"Breathing deeply is the simplest and most powerful of remedies – always within reach, yet so often overlooked."

Dr. Andrew Weil

LIVIA K.RIVERS

4-7-8 Breathing: The Secret to Calm and Focus

How to Use the 4-7-8 Technique to Reduce Anxiety and Improve Sleep

Copyright © 2024 by Livia K.Rivers

Livia K.Rivers has no responsibility for the persistence or accuracy of URLs for external or third-party Internet Websites referred to in this publication and does not guarantee that any content on such Websites is, or will remain, accurate or appropriate.

Third edition

This book was professionally typeset on Reedsy.
Find out more at reedsy.com

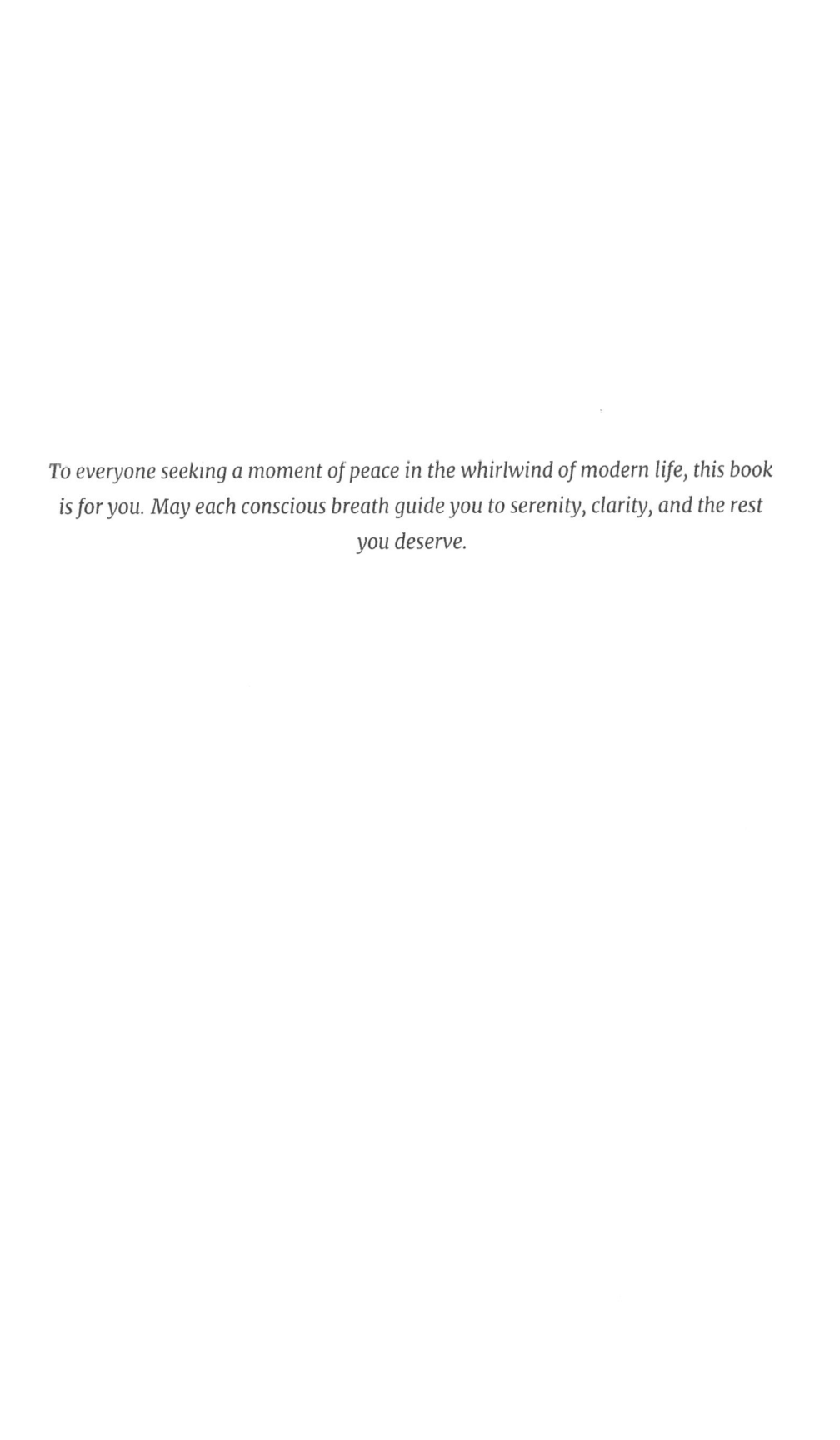

To everyone seeking a moment of peace in the whirlwind of modern life, this book is for you. May each conscious breath guide you to serenity, clarity, and the rest you deserve.

Contents

Foreword	ii
Acknowledgments	iv
Introduction	1
Chapter 1: Breathing and well-being	5
A- Anatomy of breathing	5
B- Impact of breathing on body and mind	8
Chapter 2: Discovering the 4-7-8 Technique	13
A- Origins of the technique	13
B- Concept of the technique	16
Chapter 3: How to Practice the 4-7-8 Technique	20
A- Step-by-step guide	20
B- Tips for effective practice	24
Chapter 5: Improving Sleep with the 4-7-8 Technique	30
A- Impact on sleep quality	31
B- Testimonials and case studies	36
Chapter 6: Other health benefits	41
A- Enhanced concentration and mental clarity	41
B- Other health benefits	44
Chapter 7: Frequently asked questions	50
▪☒Answers to frequently asked questions	50
Conclusion	56
Appendices	59
▪☒ Additional Resources and Tools	59
References	64
▪☒ Bibliography	64

Foreword

In today's fast-paced world, where stress and anxiety have become almost constant companions, finding a way to cultivate calm and focus is more essential than ever. Amidst the noise of modern life, the simplicity of our breath is often overlooked. Yet, within each inhale and exhale lies a profound power—a power that can transform our mental and physical well-being.

The 4-7-8 breathing technique, introduced in this book, offers a path to this transformation. Rooted in ancient practices and adapted for the demands of contemporary life, this rhythmic breathing method is not just a tool for relaxation; it is a gateway to deeper mental clarity, improved sleep, and lasting inner peace. Through its simplicity, it provides a momentary escape from the whirlwind of our thoughts and allows us to reconnect with ourselves in a meaningful way.

This book is much more than a guide to mastering a breathing technique. It is an invitation to slow down, to be present, and to reclaim control over your mind and body. As you journey through these pages, you'll discover not only the science behind the 4-7-8 method but also the stories of those who have experienced its life-changing effects.

This foreword isn't about convincing you of the importance of this practice—it's about encouraging you to explore the potential that already resides within you. Each breath you take is an opportunity to reset, to find calm in chaos, and to strengthen your focus in a distracted world.

Whether you are new to conscious breathing or looking to deepen your practice, this book will guide you every step of the way. Embrace it with an open heart and a curious mind. Your journey to a more peaceful, focused, and balanced life begins here.

Livia K.Rivers

Acknowledgments

This book would not have come to life without the support, guidance, and expertise of many individuals who generously shared their knowledge and passion for breathing techniques and mindfulness.

First, I extend my deepest gratitude to **Dr. Emily Foster** from the University of Florida, whose research on the physiological effects of breathing patterns inspired much of the content in this book. Her groundbreaking work in the field of respiratory science has been a beacon of knowledge that continues to influence so many.

I am also immensely thankful to **Dr. David Greene** at the University of Texas, who provided invaluable feedback during the writing process. His studies on stress management and breathing techniques have shed light on the profound connection between breath and emotional regulation.

To **Professor Sarah Holden** of New York University, your insights into the psychological aspects of breathing and mindfulness added depth and richness to this work. Your dedication to helping individuals find balance in a chaotic world is truly commendable, and this book is all the better for your wisdom.

A special thanks goes to **Dr. Michael Roberts** at the University of Toronto in Canada. His research into holistic health and wellness, particularly the role of breath in promoting mental clarity, has been instrumental in shaping the chapters of this book. His encouragement to bring this knowledge to a broader audience has been unwavering, and for that, I am forever grateful.

Without the contributions and support of these remarkable professionals, this book would not have seen the light of day. Their dedication to advancing the understanding of breathing techniques and their applications in everyday life is a testament to the power of collaboration and shared knowledge.

Finally, to you, the reader: I hope this book has provided you with valuable insights and practical tools for incorporating the 4-7-8 breathing method into your life. If you found this guide helpful, I kindly ask that you leave a review. Your feedback not only helps this book reach more readers but also ensures that others can benefit from the techniques and knowledge shared within its pages. Your voice matters, and it helps others discover the power of breath to transform their lives. Thank you for being a part of this journey.

Introduction

In today's fast-paced world, the need for calm has never been greater. Anxiety, stress, and sleepless nights have become unwelcome companions for so many of us. The pressures of modern life can feel overwhelming, leaving us with little time to breathe—both figuratively and literally. That's where the power of the breath comes into play. Conscious breathing, specifically the 4-7-8 technique, offers a simple yet transformative way to reclaim a sense of calm and focus.

Breathing is often taken for granted. It happens automatically, with little thought or effort. However, when approached with intention, it becomes a powerful tool for managing the mind and body. Conscious breathing taps into the body's natural mechanisms to restore balance, lower stress levels, and bring about a sense of peace. It helps anchor you in the present, offering respite from the constant buzz of worries and the relentless pace of the outside world. The 4-7-8 technique stands out because of its simplicity, accessibility, and effectiveness. It is a rhythm of breathing that promotes a profound state of relaxation by syncing the mind with the body's natural rhythms.

The beauty of conscious breathing lies in its accessibility—it's something we can all do. No special equipment, location, or training is required. All you need is a little time, a bit of practice, and a willingness to give it a try. With each mindful breath, you are not just filling your lungs with air; you are filling your body and mind with calm and clarity. Over time, this simple practice can transform your relationship with stress and anxiety, allowing you to approach life's challenges with a greater sense of ease and confidence.

The 4-7-8 technique isn't just another trend. It is rooted in ancient practices and validated by modern science. Whether you're dealing with the pressures of work, family, or the general hustle and bustle of daily life, this technique is designed to give you a moment of peace—a pause in the storm. It's a way to regain control when everything feels out of control, a method to quiet the mind when it's racing with a million thoughts. For anyone who's ever felt overwhelmed by the demands of the day, this practice offers an anchor.

What makes the 4-7-8 technique so effective? The answer lies in the deliberate rhythm of the breath. By slowing down your breathing and focusing on specific counts, you shift your nervous system out of the "fight or flight" mode that often dominates during times of stress. You tap into the parasympathetic nervous system—the body's natural "rest and digest" mode—bringing a sense of calm that washes over you like a wave of relief. This rhythmic breathing helps to reduce anxiety by regulating your body's stress response, lowering your heart rate, and calming the mind.

Many people have found this technique to be a game-changer when it comes to improving sleep. When stress and anxiety keep you up at night, the 4-7-8 method can help your mind and body unwind, making it easier to drift off to sleep and stay asleep. The technique's simplicity makes it easy to integrate into your nightly routine, allowing you to replace restless nights with deep, rejuvenating sleep.

The beauty of the 4-7-8 technique is that it works for anyone, anywhere, at any time. Whether you're sitting in traffic, lying in bed, or preparing for a big meeting, this technique is your go-to tool for finding calm in the chaos. It's an antidote to the stress that has become so prevalent in modern life, offering a simple, effective way to regain balance and inner peace.

Like many of you, I once struggled with stress and anxiety. There were

INTRODUCTION

nights when sleep felt like an elusive dream, and days when the weight of responsibilities felt overwhelming. It wasn't until I discovered the power of conscious breathing that I found a way to navigate life with more ease. The 4-7-8 technique became my lifeline—a simple practice that I could turn to whenever I needed a moment of calm. It helped me manage my anxiety, improve my sleep, and regain control over my mind and body.

This book is born out of that experience. It's for anyone who has ever felt overwhelmed, anxious, or simply in need of a moment of peace. It's for those who are looking for a way to quiet the mind, reduce stress, and improve their overall well-being. Through the 4-7-8 technique, you can reclaim your breath, and in doing so, reclaim your life.

This book is designed to be a comprehensive guide to mastering the 4-7-8 breathing technique. We will start by exploring the science behind conscious breathing and the impact it has on the body and mind. From there, we'll dive into the specifics of the 4-7-8 technique—its origins, how it works, and why it's so effective. You'll learn how to integrate this technique into your daily life, using it to reduce anxiety, improve sleep, and enhance your overall well-being.

Each chapter offers practical guidance, tips, and exercises to help you get the most out of the 4-7-8 technique. You'll also find personal stories and case studies that demonstrate the real-world impact of this practice. By the end of the book, you'll have everything you need to make conscious breathing a natural part of your daily routine.

This journey is not just about learning a new technique—it's about embracing a new way of living. A way that prioritizes calm, focus, and well-being. A way that empowers you to navigate life's challenges with greater ease and confidence. With the 4-7-8 technique, you have the tools to create lasting change in your life, one breath at a time.

As you embark on this journey, know that you are not alone. This book is here to guide you every step of the way, offering support, encouragement, and practical advice. Together, we will explore the power of conscious breathing and discover how the 4-7-8 technique can help you achieve the calm and focus you've been searching for.

Chapter 1: Breathing and well-being

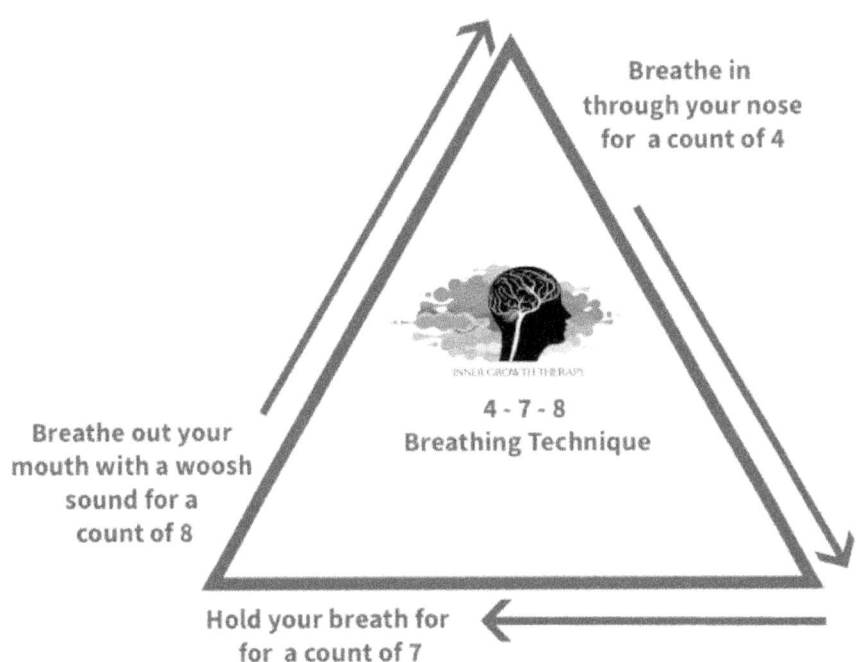

A- Anatomy of breathing

Breathing is something we do every moment of our lives, yet it often goes unnoticed. Each inhale and exhale is a rhythmic dance between our body and the world around us, but how often do we truly stop and think about this process? When we breathe consciously, we can harness the power of our breath to calm the mind and restore balance to the body. To understand the profound impact of conscious breathing, it helps to take a closer look at what's happening inside us with each breath.

The process of breathing involves much more than just filling our lungs with air. It's a complex system of muscles, nerves, and organs working together to deliver oxygen to every cell in our body while removing carbon dioxide. Understanding this process can help you appreciate the power of breath control, particularly the 4-7-8 technique, which taps into this natural system to promote relaxation and focus.

At the core of breathing lies the diaphragm, a dome-shaped muscle that sits beneath the lungs and separates the chest cavity from the abdomen. When we inhale, the diaphragm contracts and moves downward, creating more space in the chest cavity. This allows the lungs to expand, drawing in air through the nose or mouth. The air travels down the trachea, filling the lungs and inflating the alveoli—tiny air sacs where oxygen is exchanged for carbon dioxide.

The exhale is just as important as the inhale. As the diaphragm relaxes and moves upward, it pushes air out of the lungs, expelling carbon dioxide. This process, known as respiration, is automatic. It happens without any conscious thought, day in and day out. However, when we bring awareness to our breath and control the rhythm, we can influence how our body responds to stress.

In moments of anxiety, the body's natural response is to speed up breathing. This is part of the "fight or flight" response, a survival mechanism designed to help us react quickly to danger. However, in modern life, this response is often triggered by stressors that aren't life-threatening, like work deadlines or traffic jams. Rapid, shallow breathing can exacerbate feelings of anxiety, sending signals to the brain that something is wrong.

This is where the 4-7-8 breathing technique comes into play. By consciously slowing down the breath, extending the exhale, and pausing between breaths, this technique helps counteract the body's stress response. The act of controlling the breath sends a message to the brain that it's time to relax. The longer exhale stimulates the vagus nerve, which plays a key role in activating the parasympathetic nervous system—the part of the nervous system responsible for promoting calmness and rest. This creates a cascading effect throughout the body, reducing heart rate, lowering blood pressure, and promoting a sense of peace.

Breathing is the bridge between the mind and the body. When we are anxious or stressed, our breath becomes shallow and rapid. This, in turn, signals to the brain that we are in danger, even if there is no immediate threat. The brain then releases stress hormones like cortisol and adrenaline, which further heighten feelings of anxiety. It's a vicious cycle, but one that can be broken by conscious breathing.

Through practices like the 4-7-8 technique, we can actively engage the mind-body connection in a positive way. By slowing down the breath and focusing on each inhale and exhale, we can shift our body's response from stress to calm. This isn't just a psychological effect—it's a physiological one. Studies have shown that conscious breathing can reduce cortisol levels, improve heart rate variability, and even alter brainwave patterns, promoting a state of relaxation and mental clarity.

In moments of stress or overwhelm, turning to the breath can offer a grounding, centering experience. The 4-7-8 technique, with its structured rhythm, provides a sense of control when everything else feels chaotic. It's a reminder that, even when we can't control external circumstances, we can control how we respond to them. This shift in focus—from the external to the internal—can have profound effects on our well-being.

Breathing isn't just about keeping us alive; it's about enhancing the quality of our lives. When we breathe consciously, we tap into a resource that is always available to us. Whether you're dealing with anxiety, fatigue, or simply the demands of daily life, conscious breathing can help you find balance and clarity. The mind and body are intricately connected, and the breath is the key to unlocking that connection.

Take a moment to reflect on your own relationship with breath. How often do you notice your breathing throughout the day? Are there moments when your breath feels shallow or rapid? How does your body respond to stress, and how might conscious breathing help shift that response?

As you embark on this journey with the 4-7-8 technique, start by simply observing your breath. There's no need to change anything at first—just become aware of it. Notice how your body feels as you breathe in and out. Where do you feel tension? Where do you feel ease? By bringing awareness to your breath, you begin the process of reconnecting with your body and mind.

Consider setting aside a few minutes each day to focus on your breath. Whether it's first thing in the morning, during a break at work, or right before bed, this simple practice can help you cultivate a sense of calm and clarity in your daily life.

B- Impact of breathing on body and mind

Breathing is more than just a function of the lungs; it's a fundamental connection between the body and the mind. Each breath carries the potential to influence both our physical state and mental well-being. When we understand the intricate relationship between breathing and how our body and mind respond, we unlock a powerful tool for achieving calmness and clarity.

Breathing isn't just about oxygenating the blood—it's a mechanism that influences every system in our body. The quality, depth, and rhythm of your breath can directly impact how you feel, think, and react to the world around you. Conscious breathing, such as the 4-7-8 technique, uses this inherent connection to shift the nervous system from a state of stress to one of relaxation. It taps into the natural processes of the body to create a sense of balance and control.

The Nervous System and the Power of Breath

To fully appreciate the impact of conscious breathing, it's helpful to understand the role of the autonomic nervous system (ANS). The ANS regulates involuntary body functions, including heart rate, digestion, and respiratory rate. It has two primary branches: the sympathetic nervous system (SNS) and the parasympathetic nervous system (PNS).

The SNS is often referred to as the "fight or flight" system. It's activated in times of stress, preparing the body to deal with perceived threats by increasing heart rate, elevating blood pressure, and speeding up breathing. While this response is essential in dangerous situations, modern life often triggers the SNS in ways that aren't beneficial—like during moments of high anxiety or chronic stress.

On the other hand, the PNS is known as the "rest and digest" system. It works to calm the body, slowing the heart rate, reducing blood pressure, and encouraging deep, steady breathing. This system is vital for recovery, healing, and overall well-being. The 4-7-8 breathing technique actively engages the PNS, creating a state of relaxation that helps counteract the effects of stress and anxiety.

By controlling the breath, you can influence the balance between these two systems. The structured rhythm of the 4-7-8 technique—four counts of inhaling, holding for seven counts, and exhaling for eight counts—provides a natural way to stimulate the PNS, calming the body and quieting the mind. The extended exhale is particularly effective in engaging the vagus nerve, which is a key player in activating the relaxation response.

The Science of Breath and the Brain

Breathing also has a profound effect on the brain. When we breathe slowly and deeply, it sends a message to the brain that we're safe and that it's okay to relax. This signal isn't just metaphorical—it's a real, physiological process. The brain responds by reducing the production of stress hormones like cortisol and adrenaline, while promoting the release of calming neurotransmitters like gamma-aminobutyric acid (GABA).

Studies have shown that conscious breathing can influence brainwave patterns, leading to a state of relaxation similar to meditation. Slow, rhythmic breathing encourages the brain to shift from beta waves—associated with active thinking and alertness—to alpha waves, which are linked to relaxation and a calm, focused state of mind. This shift in brainwaves can improve mental clarity, reduce anxiety, and enhance overall cognitive function.

The 4-7-8 technique is particularly effective in promoting this shift. The structured counting helps quiet the mind, preventing it from wandering or getting caught up in anxious thoughts. By focusing on the rhythm of the breath, you give your mind something to anchor to, making it easier to enter a state of calm and focus.

Physical Benefits of Conscious Breathing

The benefits of conscious breathing extend beyond the brain. When we breathe deeply and slowly, it has a direct impact on our cardiovascular system. Slow breathing lowers blood pressure, reduces the heart rate, and improves circulation. This not only helps reduce the physical symptoms of stress but also promotes overall cardiovascular health.

Conscious breathing can also improve digestion. When we're stressed, the body diverts energy away from digestion and toward dealing with perceived threats. This can lead to digestive issues like bloating, indigestion, and discomfort. Engaging the parasympathetic nervous system through conscious breathing helps shift energy back to the digestive system, allowing for better nutrient absorption and a more efficient digestive process.

Additionally, deep, controlled breathing can enhance immune function. Stress is known to weaken the immune system, making us more susceptible to illness. By reducing stress through conscious breathing, we can support the body's natural defenses, helping to prevent illness and promote healing.

Reflection: The Power of Conscious Breathing in Your Life

Take a moment to consider how your own breathing patterns might be affecting your body and mind. Are there moments when you notice yourself holding your breath or breathing shallowly? How does your body feel in those moments? How does your mind respond?

As you explore the 4-7-8 technique, pay attention to the changes in your body and mind. Notice how your breath influences your heart rate, your muscle tension, and your overall sense of well-being. By tuning into these subtle shifts, you can begin to cultivate a deeper awareness of the mind-body connection and harness the power of your breath to create a sense of calm and clarity.

Incorporating conscious breathing into your daily life doesn't have to be complicated. Even a few minutes of focused breathing each day can have a profound impact on your well-being. Whether you're dealing with a stressful situation, trying to improve your focus, or simply looking to enhance your overall health, the 4-7-8 technique offers a simple, accessible way to tap into the healing power of breath.

Chapter 2: Discovering the 4-7-8 Technique

A- Origins of the technique

The 4-7-8 breathing technique, while popularized in recent years, draws on ancient wisdom rooted in the traditions of pranayama, the yogic practice of controlling the breath. In ancient India, yogis recognized the profound impact of breath on the mind and body. They discovered that by intentionally altering the breath's rhythm and depth, they could influence their mental and physical states. Over centuries, these breathing practices evolved, with different techniques emerging to address specific needs—from calming an overactive mind to energizing the body.

The 4-7-8 breathing technique has its origins in this tradition but was adapted and simplified for the modern world by Dr. Andrew Weil, a renowned physician and advocate of integrative medicine. Dr. Weil drew on his knowledge of pranayama and combined it with contemporary understandings of stress and anxiety to create a method that is both accessible and powerful.

While the technique's roots are in ancient practices, it was designed specifically to meet the needs of our fast-paced, often overwhelming modern lives.
Dr. Weil recognized that anxiety and sleep disorders are two of the most prevalent issues facing people today. With constant demands, the relentless flow of information, and the pressures of daily life, our nervous systems

are often stuck in a state of hyperarousal. This chronic activation of the sympathetic nervous system, or the "fight or flight" response, keeps us in a constant state of alertness, making it difficult to relax, focus, or sleep.

The 4-7-8 technique was tailored to counteract this overactivity. By focusing on controlled breathing, the technique helps to activate the parasympathetic nervous system—the "rest and digest" response—which allows the body and mind to relax. The simplicity of the method makes it easy to integrate into even the busiest of routines, offering a practical solution to combat stress and anxiety.

Evolution to Address Modern Stress and Sleep Issues

Over time, the 4-7-8 breathing technique evolved into a trusted tool for addressing specific issues like anxiety and insomnia. Dr. Weil noticed that by altering the breath's rhythm in a structured way—specifically through the 4-7-8 pattern—individuals could experience a marked reduction in their stress levels. The technique was designed to lengthen the exhale, which has been shown to naturally trigger the relaxation response.

The structure of the technique is deliberate. The four-count inhale fills the lungs with oxygen, energizing the body and mind. The seven-count hold allows the oxygen to fully saturate the blood, nourishing cells throughout the body. Finally, the eight-count exhale releases carbon dioxide, expelling tension and promoting relaxation. This elongated exhalation is particularly important for those suffering from anxiety, as it helps to slow the heart rate and signal the brain that it's safe to calm down.

For those dealing with insomnia, the 4-7-8 technique offers a natural way to prepare the body for rest. Many people struggle with sleep because their minds are racing with thoughts, or their bodies are still in a heightened state of alertness. By focusing on the breath and following the 4-7-8 pattern, individuals can guide their bodies into a more relaxed state, making it easier to fall asleep and stay asleep.

Why the Technique Works for Anxiety and Sleep

The success of the 4-7-8 technique in addressing anxiety and sleep issues lies in its ability to directly influence the autonomic nervous system. When we're stressed, the body enters a state of hyperarousal. The heart beats faster, breathing becomes shallow, and the mind races. These are all signs that the sympathetic nervous system is in control. While this response is useful in actual emergencies, it's detrimental when triggered by everyday stressors.

The 4-7-8 technique works by shifting control from the sympathetic nervous system to the parasympathetic nervous system. By slowing the breath and focusing on the rhythm, you engage the vagus nerve—a key component of the parasympathetic nervous system. This leads to a cascade of physiological changes: the heart rate slows, blood pressure decreases, and the body relaxes. Over time, regular practice of the 4-7-8 technique can help reset the body's baseline, making it easier to manage stress and anxiety in the long term.

This breathing technique also has a significant impact on sleep. The structured pattern of 4-7-8 helps to quiet the mind, which is often the biggest obstacle to falling asleep. Instead of being caught in a cycle of anxious thoughts, focusing on the breath creates a mental anchor that pulls attention away from racing thoughts and towards a calming rhythm. The result is a gradual shift from wakefulness to relaxation, making it easier to drift into sleep.

How Can This Technique Fit into Your Life?

Consider your current relationship with stress and sleep. Are there moments when anxiety feels overwhelming, or nights when sleep seems elusive? The 4-7-8 technique is a tool you can carry with you everywhere. It's simple enough to practice during a moment of stress at work, or while lying in bed at night struggling to fall asleep. The key is to make it a regular part of your routine.

Try incorporating the 4-7-8 technique into your daily life for the next week. Spend a few minutes each morning or evening practicing the rhythm of the breath. Pay attention to how your body responds—notice any shifts in your energy, focus, or relaxation. This simple act of conscious breathing can create profound changes in your overall well-being.

By understanding the origins and evolution of the 4-7-8 technique, you're equipped with a tool that has stood the test of time—one that is uniquely suited to address the challenges of anxiety and sleep in our modern world

B- Concept of the technique

At its core, the 4-7-8 breathing technique is a simple yet profoundly effective practice that harmonizes the rhythm of breath to foster calmness, reduce anxiety, and improve sleep. This method isn't just about regulating oxygen intake; it's about reclaiming control over your mental and physical state through something as fundamental as your breath.
   The Science Behind the 4-7-8 Technique

The 4-7-8 technique works by altering your body's autonomic nervous system. This system controls involuntary processes, such as heart rate and digestion, and is divided into two branches: the sympathetic nervous system, responsible for the "***fight or flight***" response, and the parasympathetic nervous system, which governs the "rest and digest" functions. When we experience stress or anxiety, the sympathetic nervous system takes over, increasing heart rate, tensing muscles, and speeding up our breath. This is useful in emergencies but detrimental when sustained over time due to chronic stress.

By practicing the 4-7-8 technique, you shift your body from the sympathetic mode to the parasympathetic mode. Each phase of the breath—the inhale for four counts, the hold for seven, and the exhale for eight—is designed to bring balance back to the autonomic nervous system. The extended exhale is particularly crucial because it signals the brain to relax, allowing the parasympathetic system to take the lead. This is why the technique is often described as a *"natural tranquilizer"* for the nervous system.

What makes the 4-7-8 technique so accessible is its simplicity. Unlike other breathing methods that may require specialized training or complicated sequences, this one can be done anywhere, anytime. No equipment or prior experience is necessary. All it requires is a commitment to focus on your breath for just a few minutes. In a world where stress is constant, and quick fixes are often fleeting, this technique offers a sustainable, reliable tool for emotional regulation and overall well-being.

Addressing Anxiety: Why It Works

Anxiety often arises from a feeling of being out of control. Whether it's caused by external circumstances or internal worries, the sensation of anxiety can be overwhelming. The 4-7-8 technique directly addresses this by giving you a simple, effective way to regain control—starting with your breath. As you practice the technique, the rhythmic breathing pattern activates the vagus nerve, which plays a critical role in controlling the parasympathetic nervous system. By stimulating this nerve, the 4-7-8 technique helps slow the heart rate, lower blood pressure, and create a sense of calm.

The counting pattern used in the technique also plays a psychological role in reducing anxiety. By focusing on the numbers and timing of each breath, you shift your attention away from anxious thoughts and into the present moment. This act of mindfulness helps to break the cycle of rumination, which is often at the root of anxiety. The longer exhale further enhances this effect by naturally slowing the heart rate and promoting relaxation.

This isn't just theoretical—many people have found that consistent practice of the 4-7-8 technique dramatically reduces their anxiety levels. Whether used in moments of acute stress or as a preventive measure, this method offers a tangible way to manage the physical and mental symptoms of anxiety.

Enhancing Sleep: A Natural Sleep Aid

Sleep problems often stem from an overactive mind. Whether it's racing thoughts, lingering stress from the day, or general restlessness, getting to sleep can sometimes feel like an impossible task. The 4-7-8 technique serves as a natural sleep aid by preparing the body and mind for rest.

When used before bedtime, the technique helps to quiet the mind and slow down the body's physiological processes. The gradual lengthening of each exhale signals to the body that it's time to relax, making it easier to transition from wakefulness to sleep. This is especially useful for those who struggle with insomnia or find themselves waking up in the middle of the night.

Regular practice of the 4-7-8 technique can create a consistent bedtime routine that signals to your brain that it's time to sleep. Over time, this can help to reset your circadian rhythms, making it easier to fall asleep and stay asleep. By focusing on the breath and practicing the 4-7-8 pattern, you're not just calming your mind—you're training your body to associate this practice with rest and relaxation.

Practical Application: A Daily Tool for Calmness and Focus

While the 4-7-8 technique is highly effective in addressing anxiety and improving sleep, its benefits extend far beyond these areas. This breathing method can be used throughout the day to maintain a sense of calmness and focus, even in the midst of a busy or stressful day.

The 4-7-8 technique into your daily routine, you can proactively manage stress before it spirals out of control. Whether practiced first thing in the morning to set a calm tone for the day, or during a mid-afternoon break to refocus your mind, this method can be a powerful tool for maintaining mental clarity and emotional balance.

In moments of high stress—such as before a big meeting, during a confrontation, or when facing a difficult decision—the 4-7-8 technique provides an immediate way to calm the mind and body. The more you practice, the more it becomes second nature, allowing you to access a sense of calm no matter what challenges arise.

Implementing the 4-7-8 Technique in Your Life

Take a moment to think about how you can incorporate the 4-7-8 technique into your daily routine. Is there a specific time of day when you feel most stressed or anxious? Could this technique serve as a calming ritual before bed, helping you wind down for the night? Consider setting aside just five minutes a day to practice the 4-7-8 technique, and observe how it impacts your overall well-being.

As you begin to integrate this breathing practice into your life, be patient with yourself. Like any new habit, it may take time to feel the full effects. But with consistent practice, the 4-7-8 technique can become a powerful ally in your journey toward greater calmness, focus, and overall mental health.

Chapter 3: How to Practice the 4-7-8 Technique

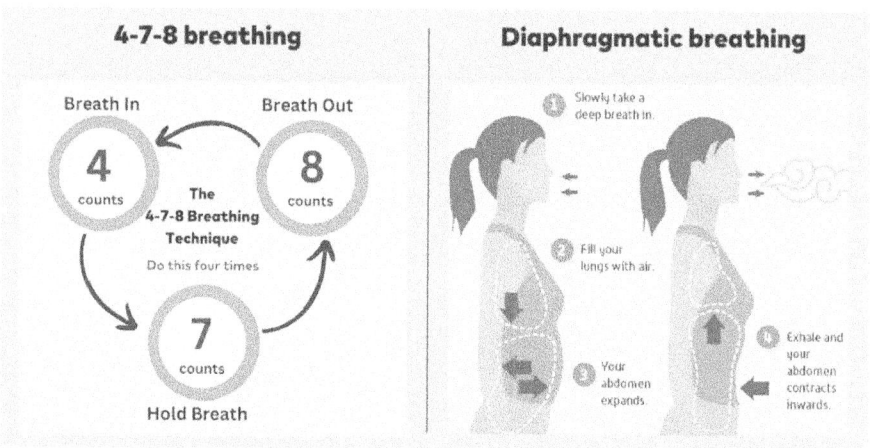

A-Step-by-step guide

The 4-7-8 breathing technique is a straightforward practice that offers profound benefits. It's ideal for beginners, but with consistency, it can also evolve into a more advanced tool for those seeking deeper relaxation, improved focus, or relief from chronic anxiety. In this section, you'll find a detailed step-by-step guide to help you master the technique and advanced tips for those who want to take their practice further.

The Basics: How to Get Started

Before diving into the advanced aspects, it's essential to grasp the core principles of the 4-7-8 technique. Here's a simple guide to help you begin:

Find a Comfortable Position: Start by sitting in a chair with your back straight or lying down in a comfortable position. If sitting, ensure that your feet are flat on the floor and your hands rest gently in your lap. You can close your eyes to block out distractions or keep them slightly open, with a soft gaze.

Exhale Completely: Begin by exhaling fully through your mouth, making a gentle whooshing sound as you push all the air out of your lungs. This helps to clear any residual tension and sets the stage for the next inhale.

Inhale for Four Counts: Close your mouth and inhale quietly through your nose for a count of four. As you breathe in, focus on drawing the air deep into your abdomen. The belly should expand outward as you fill your lungs.

Hold Your Breath for Seven Counts: After inhaling, hold your breath for a count of seven. This is where the technique starts to work its magic. Holding the breath increases the oxygen in your bloodstream and gives your body a chance to absorb it fully.

Exhale for Eight Counts: Slowly exhale completely through your mouth for a count of eight, making the same whooshing sound as you did at the start. This extended exhalation is key to activating the relaxation response in your body.

Repeat the Cycle: This is one complete breath cycle. You should repeat this cycle four times, making a total of four breaths. Initially, it's recommended to practice only these four cycles until you become more comfortable with the technique.

That's all there is to it—four cycles of 4-7-8 breathing, performed once or twice daily, is enough to begin noticing the calming effects. But once you've mastered the basics, there's room to deepen your practice.

Advanced Tips for Deepening Your Practice

As with any practice, the more you engage with the 4-7-8 technique, the more benefits you'll reap.

If you're looking to take your practice to the next level, here are some advanced tips to enhance your experience:

Extend the Practice Duration: After a few weeks of consistent practice, you may find that four breath cycles no longer feel as challenging. At this point, you can gradually increase the number of cycles to six or eight. However, it's important not to rush this process. The key to deepening your practice lies in patience and consistency, not in how many cycles you can perform at once.

Use Visualization: While practicing, you can enhance the calming effects by incorporating visualization. As you inhale, imagine drawing in a warm, golden light that fills your body with peace and calmness. When holding your breath, visualize this light settling into every cell of your body, nourishing and healing it. On the exhale, picture any tension, stress, or negative energy leaving your body as a dark mist, dissipating into the air.

Focus on Your Heart Rate: One of the key benefits of the 4-7-8 technique is its ability to slow the heart rate. For a more advanced practice, try focusing on your pulse during the breath cycle. You might notice that your heart rate increases slightly on the inhale and slows down on the exhale. By honing in on this subtle rhythm, you can deepen your awareness of your body's response to the practice.

Practice in Different Positions: While the standard position for the 4-7-8 technique is seated or lying down, you can experiment with different postures to see how they affect your practice. For example, practicing while standing with your feet shoulder-width apart and your knees slightly bent can help to ground you. Alternatively, practicing in a restorative yoga pose, such as child's pose or legs-up-the-wall, can enhance relaxation.

Incorporate the Technique into Movement: Once you're comfortable with the 4-7-8 technique, try integrating it into movement practices such as walking meditation or gentle yoga. Synchronizing your breath with your movements can create a deeper mind-body connection and help you carry the sense of calm from your practice into your daily life.

Set an Intention Before Each Practice: Before beginning your 4-7-8 breathing, take a moment to set an intention for your practice. Whether it's to release anxiety, improve focus, or simply cultivate a sense of peace, having a clear intention can enhance the effectiveness of your session. After completing the breath cycles, reflect on how well your intention was met and carry that feeling into the rest of your day.

Explore Extended Breath Holds: Once you've practiced for several months, you might feel comfortable extending the breath hold portion of the cycle. Holding the breath for up to ten counts (or even longer) can intensify the calming effects and deepen the relaxation response. However, it's important to do this gradually and listen to your body's signals. If you ever feel lightheaded or uncomfortable, return to the standard 4-7-8 count.

Combine with Meditation or Journaling: To maximize the mental clarity and emotional balance that the 4-7-8 technique offers, try combining it with other mindfulness practices. For example, after completing your breath cycles, spend a few minutes meditating on a positive affirmation or journaling about how you feel. This can help to integrate the effects of the technique into your mind and emotions, creating a more holistic sense of well-being.

Take a moment to think about how you can create a ritual around your 4-7-8 breathing practice. Is there a specific time of day when you feel most in need of a reset? Could you pair your practice with another calming activity, such as lighting a candle, playing soft music, or sipping a cup of herbal tea? By turning your practice into a ritual, you can make it a sacred part of your daily routine—something that you look forward to and that nurtures both your body and your mind.

As you deepen your practice, keep in mind that progress may be gradual. The true power of the 4-7-8 technique lies in its simplicity and consistency. With time, you'll likely notice that this method not only reduces anxiety and improves sleep but also enhances your overall sense of well-being.

B- Tips for effective practice

The 4-7-8 breathing technique may seem simple on the surface, but it holds remarkable power for transforming your mental and physical well-being. By focusing on your breath, you tap into your body's natural ability to calm the nervous system and restore balance. Whether you're a beginner or looking to deepen your practice, this section provides practical and advanced tips to maximize the benefits of the 4-7-8 technique.

Start Small and Stay Consistent
   Consistency is the foundation of any practice, and the 4-7-8 technique is no exception. Begin with just a few minutes a day. Even though it may be tempting to dive in and practice for longer periods, starting small will help your body adjust and make the practice feel more manageable. Aim to practice once or twice a day, ideally at the same time each day, to build a habit. For

many, practicing first thing in the morning or before bed works best.

Establishing a consistent routine signals to your body that this is a time to slow down, breathe deeply, and reset. Consistency also allows you to gradually experience the technique's full range of benefits, from reduced anxiety to improved sleep.

Create a Calming Environment

Creating a peaceful environment is essential to fully immersing yourself in the 4-7-8 technique. Choose a quiet space where you won't be disturbed. Turn off distractions like your phone, television, or other electronic devices. Soft lighting, gentle music, or even nature sounds can create a calming atmosphere. Consider adding elements like a cozy blanket, comfortable chair, or aromatherapy to enhance relaxation.

The environment you create around your practice helps signal to your mind and body that it's time to shift gears from the stress of daily life to a space of calm and focus. While it's not necessary to have the perfect setting every time you practice, making an effort to create a serene environment can make your practice more enjoyable and effective.

Focus on Your Breath, Not Perfection

One of the key principles of the 4-7-8 technique is focusing on your breath and the present moment. During practice, it's natural for your mind to wander, or for thoughts to pop up. The goal isn't to push those thoughts away or to expect perfection; it's to gently bring your focus back to your breath each time you notice your mind drifting.

You might find that some days your breath feels smooth and effortless, while other days it may feel more strained. This is completely normal. The point is not to force your breath or hold it too tightly. Simply allow the rhythm of your breath to guide you. Embrace the process and give yourself permission to be wherever you are that day.

Use Gentle Reminders

Sometimes, even with the best of intentions, you might forget to practice. Setting gentle reminders can be helpful. You might place a sticky note on your bathroom mirror, set an alarm on your phone, or even tie your practice to an existing habit. For example, you could practice the 4-7-8 technique right after brushing your teeth or while waiting for your morning coffee to brew.

These gentle reminders are not meant to add pressure but to support you in integrating the practice into your daily routine.

Incorporate Mindfulness

Mindfulness and conscious breathing go hand-in-hand. While practicing the 4-7-8 technique, invite mindfulness into the experience. Pay attention to the sensation of your breath entering and leaving your body. Notice how your abdomen rises with each inhale and falls with each exhale. Feel the cool air as it enters your nostrils and the warmth as you exhale through your mouth.

By staying mindful, you bring awareness to the present moment, helping to anchor your attention and deepen your relaxation. Practicing mindfulness during your 4-7-8 sessions can also make it easier to access this state of calmness and focus in other areas of your life.

Adjust the Technique to Fit Your Needs

One of the beautiful aspects of the 4-7-8 technique is its adaptability. If you find the breath counts challenging at first, it's okay to modify them slightly. You might start with a 3-6-7 rhythm until you feel comfortable extending to the full 4-7-8 cycle. The most important thing is to find a rhythm that feels natural and sustainable for you.

Additionally, there may be times when holding your breath for seven counts feels too intense. In these moments, listen to your body and adjust as needed. The purpose of the 4-7-8 technique is to promote relaxation, not to create stress or strain. By honoring your body's signals, you'll ensure that your practice remains both effective and enjoyable.

Incorporate the Technique into Daily Life

While setting aside dedicated time for the 4-7-8 technique is important, you can also weave it into your everyday activities. Practice while waiting in line, during a stressful commute, or in moments of anxiety or overwhelm. The beauty of this technique is that it can be done almost anywhere, allowing you to reset and regain calmness throughout the day.

Imagine you're sitting in traffic, feeling your stress levels rise. Instead of letting frustration take over, you can use the 4-7-8 technique to soothe your nervous system. By integrating the practice into your daily life, you'll find that it becomes a reliable tool for navigating challenges with greater ease.

Advanced Tips for Deepening Your Practice

Once you've established a consistent practice, you may want to explore deeper aspects of the 4-7-8 technique.

Here are some advanced tips for taking your practice to the next level:

Extend the Breath Hold: With time and practice, you may feel comfortable extending the breath hold beyond seven counts. Gradually increase the hold to eight, nine, or even ten counts, allowing your body to absorb more oxygen and deepen your relaxation. Be mindful to listen to your body, and don't push yourself beyond your limits.

Incorporate Visualization: During the breath hold, visualize a wave of calmness spreading throughout your body. Imagine this wave washing away tension, anxiety, and stress with each exhale. Visualization can amplify the technique's effects, making it even more potent in reducing anxiety and promoting relaxation.

Practice with a Focus on Heart Rate: As you progress, start paying attention to your heart rate during the 4-7-8 cycles. Notice how your heart rate slows during the breath hold and exhale. This awareness helps deepen the mind-body connection and can be a powerful tool for managing stress and anxiety.

Practice in Different Settings: Experiment with practicing in various environments to see how the technique impacts your state of mind. Try practicing outdoors in nature, in a quiet room with soft lighting, or even during a walk. Different settings can offer unique benefits, helping you find the optimal environment for your practice.

Combine with Meditation: For those looking to further deepen their relaxation and mental clarity, combining the 4-7-8 technique with meditation can be incredibly effective. Start with a few rounds of the 4-7-8 breathing, then transition into a mindfulness meditation, focusing on your breath or a mantra. This combination can enhance both practices, leaving you feeling more grounded and centered.

Journal After Practice: Journaling after your practice can be a powerful way to process and reflect on your experience. Take a few minutes to jot down how you feel, any insights you gained, or anything that came up during your session. This practice of self-reflection can help reinforce the positive effects of the technique and create a deeper sense of connection with your breath.

As you continue your journey with the 4-7-8 technique, it's important to cultivate patience. Results may not be immediate, but with consistent practice, you will notice shifts in your anxiety levels, sleep patterns, and overall sense of well-being. Trust the process and allow yourself to grow into the practice at your own pace.

Take a moment after each session to reflect on your experience. How does your body feel? What emotions are present? By acknowledging these observations, you strengthen your connection with the practice and encourage long-term growth.

The 4-7-8 technique is a lifelong tool for promoting calmness, focus, and relaxation. Whether you're just starting or deepening your practice, these tips will help you maximize the benefits and create a sustainable, nurturing routine.

Chapter 5: Improving Sleep with the 4-7-8 Technique

The 478 Breathing Technique

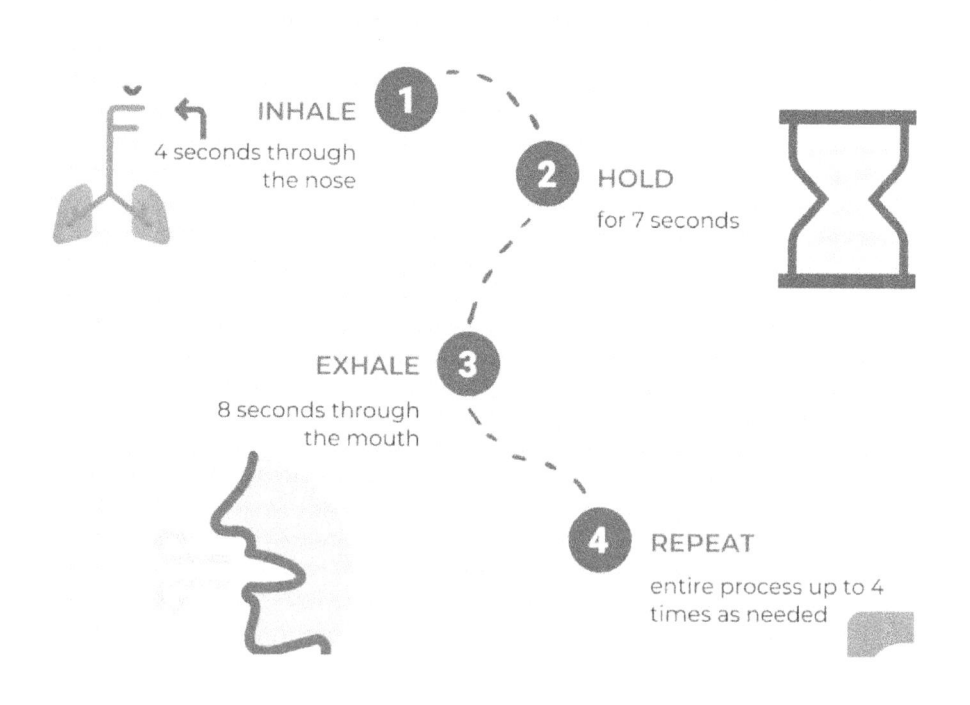

1 INHALE — 4 seconds through the nose

2 HOLD — for 7 seconds

3 EXHALE — 8 seconds through the mouth

4 REPEAT — entire process up to 4 times as needed

CHAPTER 5: IMPROVING SLEEP WITH THE 4-7-8 TECHNIQUE

A-Impact on sleep quality

The quality of sleep profoundly affects every aspect of our lives, from how we feel emotionally to our cognitive performance and physical health. In a world where sleep disorders and restless nights have become alarmingly common, it's vital to understand how the simple act of breathing can directly influence our sleep patterns and help us achieve restorative rest. The 4-7-8 breathing technique is not just a relaxation tool; it's a sleep-enhancing practice that addresses the root of many sleep issues, such as stress, anxiety, and an overactive mind.

To fully grasp the power of this technique on sleep, let's explore the science of sleep patterns and how rhythmic breathing directly impacts them.

Understanding Sleep Patterns
   Sleep is not a single, uniform experience; it's a complex cycle composed of different stages, each playing a crucial role in restoring and rejuvenating the body and mind. These stages fall into two primary categories: **non-rapid eye movement (NREM) sleep** and **rapid eye movement (REM) sleep**.

Understanding how breathing influences these stages can illuminate the 4-7-8 technique's profound impact on sleep quality.

- **Stage 1 (NREM):** This is the lightest stage of sleep, where you drift in and out of wakefulness. Your breathing begins to slow, your heart rate decreases, and your muscles start to relax. It's a transitional stage, setting the stage for deeper sleep.
- **Stage 2 (NREM):** In this stage, your body temperature drops, and your breathing becomes even more rhythmic. This stage accounts for the majority of your sleep cycle and prepares your body for the deep sleep that follows.

- **Stage 3 (NREM):** Also known as deep sleep or slow-wave sleep, this stage is essential for physical restoration. Your breathing is at its slowest and most regular during this phase. It's also the time when your body repairs tissues, builds bone and muscle, and strengthens the immune system.
- **REM Sleep:** This is the dream stage, characterized by rapid eye movements and increased brain activity. During REM sleep, your breathing becomes irregular, similar to when you're awake. This stage is crucial for cognitive functions like memory and learning.

For optimal health, you need to cycle through all these stages multiple times during the night. However, stress and anxiety can disrupt this natural progression, leading to fragmented sleep. An overactive mind can keep you in the lighter stages of sleep, preventing you from reaching the deep, restorative stages.

This is where the 4-7-8 breathing technique comes into play.

How the 4-7-8 Technique Influences Sleep Patterns

The 4-7-8 breathing technique works on multiple levels to enhance sleep quality. At its core, it directly engages your parasympathetic nervous system—the part of your nervous system responsible for the "rest and digest" response. By activating this system, you counteract the "fight or flight" response that stress and anxiety trigger, which often keeps you tossing and turning at night.

Slowing Down the Breath for Deeper Relaxation

The deliberate pattern of inhaling for four counts, holding for seven counts, and exhaling for eight counts mimics the natural breathing rhythm your body experiences during deep sleep. When you practice this technique, you send a signal to your brain that it's time to slow down, relax, and transition into sleep. The prolonged exhalation is particularly important because it encourages the release of carbon dioxide from the body, which lowers your heart rate and blood pressure, setting the stage for deeper rest.

Reducing the Activity of the Sympathetic Nervous System

Stress and anxiety trigger the sympathetic nervous system, which is responsible for the fight-or-flight response. This response increases your heart rate, quickens your breathing, and floods your body with stress hormones like cortisol. When this system is activated at night, it becomes challenging to fall asleep or stay asleep. The 4-7-8 technique helps shift your body from this hyper-alert state to a more relaxed, parasympathetic state, where sleep becomes more accessible.

Calming the Overactive Mind

Racing thoughts are a common barrier to falling asleep. Whether you're replaying the events of the day, worrying about tomorrow, or feeling overwhelmed by life's pressures, an overactive mind can keep you lying awake for hours. The 4-7-8 technique provides a focal point—your breath—that helps anchor your attention and quiet mental chatter. By focusing on the rhythm of your breathing, you shift your awareness away from intrusive thoughts and towards a calming, repetitive action, making it easier to drift into sleep.

Promoting a Sense of Control

Sleep problems can create a sense of helplessness. The more you struggle to sleep, the more anxious you become about not sleeping, creating a vicious cycle. The 4-7-8 technique offers a sense of control over your body's relaxation process. By practicing this technique, you take an active role in calming your mind and preparing your body for sleep, which can significantly reduce the anxiety around falling asleep.

Practical Tips for Using the 4-7-8 Technique to Improve Sleep

While the 4-7-8 technique is effective on its own, combining it with other sleep-enhancing practices can amplify its benefits.

Here are some practical tips for integrating the technique into your bedtime routine:

Establish a Relaxing Pre-Sleep Ritual:
Creating a consistent bedtime routine can signal to your body that it's time to wind down. Activities like reading a book, taking a warm bath, or practicing gentle stretches can help prepare your mind and body for sleep. Incorporating the 4-7-8 technique into this routine can further deepen your relaxation.

Practice in Bed:
The beauty of the 4-7-8 technique is that it can be practiced anywhere, but doing it in bed right before sleep can be especially effective. Lie comfortably on your back or side, close your eyes, and begin the breathing cycle. As you practice, visualize yourself sinking deeper into your mattress with each exhale, releasing any tension or stress.

Combine with Visualization or Affirmations:
Pairing the 4-7-8 technique with positive visualization or affirmations can enhance its calming effects. For example, while holding your breath for seven counts, you might imagine a soothing wave of relaxation spreading through your body. Or, as you exhale for eight counts, silently repeat a calming affirmation, such as *"I am at peace"* or *"My mind is calm."*

Use It During Nighttime Awakenings:
Waking up in the middle of the night is a common sleep issue, and getting back to sleep can sometimes feel impossible. If you find yourself awake during the night, practicing the 4-7-8 technique can help you return to a relaxed state and drift back to sleep more quickly.

Pair It with Aromatherapy:
Scents like lavender, chamomile, and sandalwood are known for their calming properties. Diffusing these essential oils in your bedroom while

practicing the 4-7-8 technique can create an even more relaxing environment, helping to ease you into sleep.

Keep Practicing Even When Sleep Improves:

The effects of the 4-7-8 technique are cumulative, meaning the more you practice, the more your body becomes conditioned to relax. Even after your sleep quality improves, continuing the practice can help maintain these benefits and prevent future sleep disruptions.

Improving sleep quality is not always an overnight process. It requires patience, consistency, and a willingness to experiment with different techniques. The 4-7-8 breathing technique offers a powerful tool for reclaiming restful nights, but it's essential to approach it with a spirit of curiosity and self-compassion. Some nights may be more challenging than others, and that's okay. Each time you practice, you're teaching your body and mind how to relax and reset.

Take a few moments after your practice to reflect on how your body feels and how your mind has shifted. Celebrate the small victories, whether it's falling asleep faster, staying asleep longer, or waking up feeling more refreshed. These are all signs that your body is responding to the practice and moving towards a state of balance.

By integrating the 4-7-8 technique into your sleep routine, you're not only improving the quality of your rest but also nurturing your overall well-being. Sleep is the foundation upon which we build our days, and with this technique, you have the power to strengthen that foundation, one breath at a time.

B- Testimonials and case studies

The transformative power of the 4-7-8 breathing technique isn't just a theory backed by scientific principles. It's a lived experience for countless individuals who have embraced this simple yet effective method to improve their sleep and overall well-being. Sharing personal stories and case studies highlights how this technique can be a beacon of hope for those struggling with anxiety, insomnia, or restless nights. These real-life examples illustrate the profound impact of rhythmic breathing on sleep patterns and demonstrate how the 4-7-8 technique can make a significant difference.

A Story of Renewal: Emily's Journey with 4-7-8 Breathing

Emily, a 35-year-old working mother of two, had been struggling with sleep for years. Between balancing her demanding job and caring for her young children, her nights were filled with stress and racing thoughts. She would often find herself staring at the ceiling at 2 AM, her mind replaying the events of the day and worrying about the next. Sleep had become elusive, and the lack of rest was taking a toll on her mental and physical health.

Emily had tried everything from sleep aids to meditation apps, but nothing seemed to work. She felt trapped in a cycle of sleeplessness, unable to break free. Then, a friend introduced her to the 4-7-8 breathing technique. Initially skeptical, Emily decided to give it a try, thinking that she had nothing to lose.

On her first night practicing the technique, she followed the simple steps: inhaling for four counts, holding her breath for seven, and exhaling slowly for eight counts. To her surprise, she felt a sense of calm wash over her body. Her heart rate slowed, and her mind began to quiet. Within minutes, she drifted off to sleep.

Over the next few weeks, Emily continued practicing the 4-7-8 technique every night before bed. She noticed a significant improvement in her sleep quality. She was falling asleep faster, staying asleep longer, and waking up feeling more refreshed. The technique had become a lifeline, helping her reclaim the restful nights she had been missing for so long.

Emily's experience is just one example of how the 4-7-8 technique can make a profound difference in someone's sleep patterns. By calming the nervous system and reducing the mental chatter that often keeps us awake, this practice creates an environment where sleep can naturally unfold.

The Science Behind the Success

Understanding the Impact on Sleep Patterns

To understand why rhythmic breathing like the 4-7-8 technique is so effective, it helps to look at how it influences sleep patterns. Sleep is a complex process, governed by both physiological and psychological factors. When the body is stressed or the mind is overactive, it disrupts the delicate balance needed for restorative sleep.

The 4-7-8 technique works by directly engaging the parasympathetic nervous system, which helps regulate the body's relaxation response. This system is responsible for calming the body and preparing it for sleep. When you practice the 4-7-8 technique, you activate this system, which slows your heart rate, reduces blood pressure, and promotes a sense of calm.

In addition to its physiological effects, the 4-7-8 technique also has a psychological impact. By focusing on your breath, you divert your attention away from stressful thoughts and towards the present moment. This mindfulness aspect of the practice helps quiet the mind, making it easier to drift into sleep.

Case studies have shown that individuals who struggle with insomnia or anxiety-related sleep disturbances often experience significant improvements in sleep quality after incorporating the 4-7-8 technique into their bedtime routine. By creating a sense of calm in both the body and mind, this practice helps restore the natural sleep cycle, allowing individuals to experience deeper, more restorative rest.

Case Study: Mark's Transformation from Sleeplessness to Serenity

Mark, a 42-year-old entrepreneur, had always been a high achiever. He thrived on the adrenaline of running his own business, but the constant pressure had taken a toll on his sleep. For years, Mark had been surviving on just a few hours of restless sleep each night. He would wake up multiple times, his mind racing with thoughts about work, and by morning, he felt exhausted and irritable.

Mark's lack of sleep began to affect his performance at work and his relationships at home. He knew something had to change, but he wasn't sure where to start. After reading about the 4-7-8 technique, he decided to give it a try.

The first few nights of practice were challenging for Mark. He found it difficult to slow down his breath and focus on the rhythm. However, he persisted, reminding himself that change takes time. Gradually, he began to notice small improvements. His mind felt less cluttered before bed, and he was able to fall asleep more quickly.

After a month of consistent practice, Mark experienced a significant transformation. He was sleeping through the night without waking up, and he felt more refreshed in the morning. His anxiety levels had decreased, and he was able to approach his work with a clearer mind. The 4-7-8 technique had not only improved his sleep but also his overall well-being.

Mark's story is a powerful testament to the effectiveness of the 4-7-8 technique. It highlights the importance of consistency and patience in the journey towards better sleep. For many people like Mark, the practice becomes more than just a tool for sleep—it becomes a pathway to a calmer, more focused life.

A Deeper Dive into the Mind-Body Connection

What makes the 4-7-8 technique so unique is its ability to bridge the gap between the mind and body. Sleep disturbances are often the result of a disconnect between these two aspects of our being. The mind races, while the body struggles to relax, creating a cycle of wakefulness that can be difficult to break.

By consciously regulating your breath, you create a direct line of communication between the mind and body. Each inhale and exhale serves as a reminder to both that it's time to rest. Over time, this practice can rewire the brain's response to stress and anxiety, making it easier to slip into a state of relaxation when it's time for sleep.

Research has shown that rhythmic breathing practices like the 4-7-8 technique can lead to changes in brainwave patterns. Specifically, it promotes the production of alpha waves, which are associated with relaxation and a calm mental state. By increasing the presence of these waves, the practice helps create the ideal conditions for sleep.

The stories and case studies shared in this chapter are just a glimpse into the potential of the 4-7-8 breathing technique to transform sleep patterns and enhance overall well-being. Whether you're struggling with chronic insomnia, occasional restless nights, or simply seeking to improve your sleep quality, this practice offers a powerful tool for change.

As you continue your journey with the 4-7-8 technique, take time to reflect on your own experience. How has the practice affected your sleep? What changes have you noticed in your body and mind? Embrace each small victory and recognize that this is a process—a journey towards a more peaceful, restorative sleep.

The 4-7-8 technique into your daily routine, you're taking a proactive step towards reclaiming your nights and nurturing your well-being. And just like Emily, Mark, and countless others, you have the potential to experience the transformative power of breath, one inhale and exhale at a time.

Chapter 6: Other health benefits

A-Enhanced concentration and mental clarity

The practice of 4-7-8 breathing isn't only about reducing anxiety or improving sleep—it also has profound effects on concentration and mental clarity. In today's world, where distractions are endless and focus is constantly being pulled in different directions, the ability to maintain mental clarity is a superpower. This chapter explores how the 4-7-8 technique can help cultivate that superpower, enhancing concentration and mental sharpness in ways that may surprise you.

The Science of Focus: How Breathing Influences Mental Clarity

At first glance, it may seem surprising that something as simple as breathing could have a significant impact on concentration. Yet, when examined closely, the link between breath and mental clarity is clear. Our breath is intimately connected with our nervous system, and our nervous system, in turn, influences cognitive function.

When you are stressed or anxious, your body goes into a "fight or flight" mode. In this state, your sympathetic nervous system is activated, flooding your body with adrenaline and cortisol. These stress hormones prepare you for immediate action, but they also reduce your ability to think clearly and make rational decisions. Your mind becomes consumed with survival, pushing out more nuanced cognitive functions like concentration and problem-solving.

By practicing the 4-7-8 technique, you engage the parasympathetic nervous system, which counters the effects of the stress response. This calms your body and mind, reducing the levels of stress hormones in your bloodstream and allowing for greater cognitive function. The clarity that follows is like a fog lifting from your mind, enabling you to think more clearly, process information more effectively, and maintain focus for longer periods.

A Deeper Look: How Breathing Sharpens the Mind

Breathwork like the 4-7-8 technique directly influences brainwave patterns, which play a significant role in mental clarity. Our brains operate on different frequencies depending on our state of mind—alpha waves, for example, are associated with a relaxed and focused mental state. When you practice the 4-7-8 technique, you promote the production of these alpha waves, which are crucial for concentration and mental sharpness.

In addition to brainwaves, oxygen levels in the brain also play a key role in cognitive function. Every time you inhale deeply, you increase the flow of oxygen to your brain. This boost of oxygen is like fuel for your brain cells, allowing them to operate at their highest capacity. With better oxygenation, your brain can work more efficiently, leading to enhanced concentration, quicker mental processing, and greater clarity in your thoughts.

It's not just about focusing harder—it's about focusing smarter. When your mind is calm and your brain is well-oxygenated, you can direct your attention more effectively. Instead of battling distractions or feeling mentally scattered, you can channel your energy into the task at hand, whether it's solving a complex problem at work or simply being present in a conversation.

CHAPTER 6: OTHER HEALTH BENEFITS

The Role of Mindfulness in Mental Clarity

The 4-7-8 breathing technique isn't just a mechanical process of inhaling, holding, and exhaling—it also encourages mindfulness. Mindfulness, the practice of bringing your attention to the present moment without judgment, is a key component in enhancing mental clarity.

When practicing the 4-7-8 technique, you naturally become more mindful of your breath. This focus on the present moment helps quiet the mental noise that often clouds our minds. Mindfulness helps reduce the overwhelming barrage of thoughts that distract us, allowing for a more focused and clear mental state.

By cultivating mindfulness through the 4-7-8 technique, you create mental space. In that space, you can think more clearly, make decisions with greater confidence, and engage with the world around you more fully. This clarity extends beyond just moments of focused work—it permeates your entire life, helping you approach challenges with a calm and steady mind.

Stories of Transformation: Real-Life Experiences with Mental Clarity

Numerous individuals have shared how the 4-7-8 breathing technique has transformed their ability to focus and think clearly. Take, for instance, Sara, a graduate student who had been struggling with overwhelming amounts of information and deadlines. After incorporating the 4-7-8 technique into her daily routine, Sara found that she was able to approach her studies with a clearer mind. She was no longer bogged down by mental fatigue or racing thoughts. Instead, she could focus on her work with renewed concentration and efficiency.

Then there's James, a software engineer who often found his mind scattered during meetings. His thoughts would drift, and he struggled to stay present.

After learning the 4-7-8 technique, James began practicing it before meetings and whenever he felt his mind wandering. The difference was remarkable—his ability to focus improved, and he was able to contribute more effectively to discussions. The technique had given him the mental clarity he needed to stay sharp and engaged.

These stories highlight how the 4-7-8 technique isn't just about relaxation—it's about empowering your mind to operate at its best. Whether you're studying for exams, solving complex problems, or simply trying to stay present in daily life, the 4-7-8 technique can provide the mental clarity you need to succeed.

Mental clarity is one of the greatest gifts we can give ourselves. It allows us to move through life with greater purpose, make better decisions, and fully engage with the world around us. The 4-7-8 breathing technique offers a simple yet powerful way to enhance that clarity, helping us navigate our lives with a calm and focused mind.

Take a moment to reflect on your own experiences with mental clarity. Have there been times when you felt mentally scattered or overwhelmed? How might the 4-7-8 technique help bring more focus and clarity into your life? As you continue your journey with this practice, embrace the mental sharpness that comes with each breath. You have the power to clear away the mental fog and create a mind that is calm, focused, and ready for whatever challenges come your way.

B- Other health benefits

The 4-7-8 breathing technique has become renowned for its ability to reduce anxiety and improve sleep, but its benefits extend far beyond these two areas. This simple yet powerful practice has a profound effect on the overall health of the body and mind. As we delve deeper into the wide-ranging health advantages of 4-7-8 breathing, it becomes clear that this technique is not just a tool for relaxation; it's a holistic practice that can transform your well-being in numerous ways.

Strengthening the Immune System

One of the lesser-known benefits of 4-7-8 breathing is its positive impact on the immune system. When stress is chronic, the body's immune response becomes suppressed, leaving us vulnerable to illness and disease. This occurs because prolonged stress elevates cortisol levels, which in turn reduces the activity of immune cells. By regularly engaging in 4-7-8 breathing, the parasympathetic nervous system is activated, which helps lower cortisol levels and promote relaxation. This shift allows the immune system to function more effectively, enhancing the body's natural defenses.

Moreover, the deep, rhythmic breathing pattern of 4-7-8 helps to oxygenate the blood, which is crucial for immune health. Oxygen-rich blood nourishes the cells and tissues, keeping them healthy and robust. When your body is well-oxygenated, it is better equipped to fight off infections and recover more quickly from illness. In this way, the 4-7-8 technique acts as a preventative health measure, supporting your immune system so that it can protect you from the inside out.

Lowering Blood Pressure

High blood pressure, or hypertension, is a common condition that affects millions of people. It's often referred to as a "silent killer" because it can lead to serious health problems like heart disease and stroke without showing any noticeable symptoms. The 4-7-8 breathing technique is a powerful ally in the fight against high blood pressure. By encouraging the body to relax, this breathing pattern helps to dilate blood vessels and improve circulation, which in turn reduces blood pressure.

Research has shown that deep, controlled breathing can lower systolic and diastolic blood pressure by reducing the activity of the sympathetic nervous system—the part of the nervous system responsible for the "fight or flight" response. By calming this response, the heart rate slows down, and blood pressure naturally decreases. For those who struggle with hypertension, incorporating 4-7-8 breathing into their daily routine can be a simple yet effective way to manage their condition and reduce the risk of serious health complications.

Enhancing Digestion

Digestive health is another area where the 4-7-8 technique can make a significant difference. Stress has a profound impact on digestion, often leading to issues such as indigestion, bloating, and irritable bowel syndrome (IBS). When the body is in a state of stress, digestion slows down or even halts altogether, as energy is diverted to more immediate survival needs. This can lead to chronic digestive problems that not only affect physical comfort but also overall health.

By activating the parasympathetic nervous system, 4-7-8 breathing helps to restore the body's "rest and digest" mode. In this state, digestion is optimized, and the body can more effectively break down and absorb nutrients. The rhythmic nature of the breathing technique also helps to massage the internal organs, promoting healthy digestion and alleviating issues like constipation and bloating. For those struggling with digestive discomfort, practicing 4-7-8 breathing before meals or during times of stress can help reset the body and support better digestive function.

Alleviating Chronic Pain

Chronic pain can be debilitating, affecting every aspect of life, from mobility to mood. The 4-7-8 breathing technique offers a natural and non-invasive way to manage chronic pain by promoting relaxation and reducing the perception of pain. When the body is tense and stressed, pain signals are amplified, making discomfort feel more intense. By calming the nervous system through 4-7-8 breathing, the body's response to pain is reduced, making it easier to cope with chronic pain conditions.

Furthermore, the deep relaxation induced by this breathing pattern can help to release tension in the muscles, which is often a contributing factor to pain. For individuals dealing with conditions like fibromyalgia, arthritis, or back pain, incorporating 4-7-8 breathing into their daily routine can offer relief and improve their quality of life. It's important to note that while this technique may not eliminate pain entirely, it can significantly reduce its impact, making it a valuable tool for pain management.

Boosting Mental Resilience

In addition to its physical health benefits, 4-7-8 breathing also plays a key role in boosting mental resilience. In today's fast-paced world, maintaining mental health is just as important as caring for the body. Chronic stress, anxiety, and emotional upheaval can take a toll on mental well-being, leaving individuals feeling drained and overwhelmed. The 4-7-8 technique offers a way to build mental resilience by calming the mind and creating space for reflection and healing.

By practicing 4-7-8 breathing regularly, you can develop a greater sense of control over your thoughts and emotions. This increased awareness allows you to respond to challenges with more clarity and calm, rather than reacting impulsively. The technique also encourages mindfulness, which can help you stay grounded in the present moment, rather than being consumed by worries about the past or future. Over time, this practice can lead to greater emotional stability and a more resilient mindset, enabling you to navigate life's ups and downs with greater ease.

Supporting Heart Health

Cardiovascular health is closely linked to stress levels, and chronic stress is a major risk factor for heart disease. The 4-7-8 breathing technique offers a way to protect your heart by reducing stress and promoting relaxation. When you practice this breathing pattern, your heart rate slows down, and your blood vessels relax, which helps to improve circulation and reduce the strain on your heart. This can lower your risk of developing heart disease and other cardiovascular conditions.

In addition to lowering blood pressure, 4-7-8 breathing can also help to balance cholesterol levels and reduce inflammation in the body—both of which are important for heart health. By incorporating this technique into your daily routine, you can support your cardiovascular system and protect your heart from the damaging effects of stress.

Elevating Mood and Promoting Emotional Well-Being

Emotional well-being is another area where the 4-7-8 breathing technique can have a significant impact. By calming the nervous system and promoting relaxation, this technique can help to alleviate symptoms of depression, anxiety, and mood swings. Deep, rhythmic breathing stimulates the release of endorphins—those "feel-good" hormones that boost mood and promote a sense of well-being.

Moreover, by practicing 4-7-8 breathing regularly, you can develop a greater sense of emotional balance. The technique encourages mindfulness, which can help you to process emotions in a healthier way. Instead of being overwhelmed by feelings of stress, anger, or sadness, you can approach these emotions with a sense of calm and clarity. Over time, this practice can lead to greater emotional stability and a more positive outlook on life.

The 4-7-8 breathing technique offers so much more than just relief from anxiety and better sleep. It has the potential to transform your health in countless ways, from boosting your immune system to enhancing mental clarity, improving digestion, managing chronic pain, and supporting cardiovascular health. This practice is a holistic tool for well-being, offering benefits that reach far beyond the immediate effects of relaxation.

Take a moment to reflect on the broader impact that 4-7-8 breathing could have on your health. How might this simple practice help you address health challenges you've been facing? What changes could you see in your physical, mental, and emotional well-being as you continue to incorporate this technique into your daily life?

As you move forward on your journey with 4-7-8 breathing, embrace the full spectrum of health benefits that this practice offers. Whether you're looking to improve your physical health, enhance your mental resilience, or simply create more balance in your life, this technique has the power to support you every step of the way.

Chapter 7: Frequently asked questions

▪️❓Answers to frequently asked questions

In every journey, there are moments when questions arise, doubts surface, and clarity is sought. With a technique as powerful as the 4-7-8 breathing method, it's natural to want to know more—whether it's understanding how to maximize its benefits, troubleshooting common challenges, or addressing any uncertainties that may linger. In this chapter, you'll find answers to some of the most frequently asked questions about the 4-7-8 technique. The goal is to provide you with deeper insight, dispel any concerns, and equip you with the knowledge needed to make this practice truly transformative.

1. How long should I practice the 4-7-8 technique each day to see results?

There isn't a strict time requirement for practicing 4-7-8 breathing, and that's one of the beauties of this method. You'll start to notice benefits—such as a sense of calm, reduced anxiety, and improved focus—within just a few sessions. However, consistency is key. Ideally, aim to practice the technique at least twice a day, once in the morning to set the tone for your day and once in the evening to help unwind before sleep. Each session only takes a couple of minutes, so it's easy to fit into even the busiest schedules.

For those seeking deeper results, such as improved sleep quality or long-term reduction in anxiety, extending your practice to three or four times a day can be beneficial. The more frequently you engage in this rhythmic breathing, the more attuned your body becomes to its calming effects. Over time, your nervous system will learn to shift more effortlessly into a state of relaxation, allowing you to access calm and clarity in even the most stressful situations.

2. Can 4-7-8 breathing help with chronic anxiety or is it just for momentary stress relief?

The 4-7-8 breathing technique is versatile enough to address both acute stress and chronic anxiety. For immediate stress relief, such as calming your nerves before a big presentation or winding down after a hectic day, this technique can bring almost instant results. The act of focusing on your breath and engaging in this structured pattern creates a pause that interrupts the cycle of stress and anxiety.

When it comes to chronic anxiety, regular practice of 4-7-8 breathing can create profound and lasting changes in how you experience and manage anxiety. Chronic anxiety often stems from a prolonged state of heightened arousal in the nervous system. By consistently practicing this technique, you help to rewire your body's stress response, making it easier to shift into a state of calm and reducing the overall intensity and frequency of anxious episodes. Over time, this can lead to a significant decrease in chronic anxiety levels, allowing you to approach life with more ease and resilience.

3. Will 4-7-8 breathing work for me if I have trouble focusing?

Difficulty focusing is something many people struggle with, especially in today's fast-paced, technology-driven world. The 4-7-8 breathing technique can be a powerful tool in helping to improve focus and concentration. By engaging in this rhythmic breathing pattern, you bring your attention away from distractions and into the present moment. The act of counting during each breath cycle creates an anchor for your mind, giving it something to hold onto, which in turn reduces mental chatter.

If focusing during the practice feels challenging at first, don't be discouraged. It's completely normal for the mind to wander, especially if you're new to mindfulness techniques. Start by gently guiding your focus back to the counting and the sensation of your breath whenever you notice your mind drifting. Over time, this process of refocusing will become easier, and you'll find that the practice not only enhances your concentration during the breathing exercise but also spills over into other areas of your life, making it easier to focus on tasks, conversations, and goals.

4. Can the 4-7-8 technique be done in any position, or do I need to be seated or lying down?

The beauty of 4-7-8 breathing is its adaptability. This technique can be practiced in any position—whether you're seated, lying down, standing, or even walking. That said, it's generally easier to begin the practice in a seated or lying-down position, especially if you're new to the technique. These positions allow you to fully relax and engage your diaphragm, which is essential for deep, effective breathing.

Once you're comfortable with the technique, feel free to experiment with practicing it in different positions throughout your day. For example, you can engage in 4-7-8 breathing while walking in nature, standing in line, or even during a brief break at work. The more you integrate this technique into various aspects of your daily routine, the more accessible its benefits will become.

5. Is it possible to overdo 4-7-8 breathing?

As with any practice, it's important to listen to your body and respect your limits. While the 4-7-8 breathing technique is generally safe for most people, doing it excessively or forcing the breath can lead to discomfort or lightheadedness, especially for beginners. Start with a few cycles—three to four repetitions—and gradually increase the number as you become more comfortable with the technique.

If at any point you feel lightheaded or uncomfortable, pause the practice and return to your normal breathing. With time, your lung capacity will improve, and you'll find it easier to engage in longer sessions without any adverse effects. The key is to approach the practice with gentleness and patience, allowing your body to adapt naturally to the rhythm of the breath.

6. Can 4-7-8 breathing be combined with other relaxation techniques?

Absolutely. The 4-7-8 breathing technique can be a powerful complement to other relaxation practices, such as meditation, yoga, or progressive muscle relaxation. Combining these techniques can enhance the overall effects, creating a more profound sense of calm and well-being. For example, you might begin a meditation session with a few cycles of 4-7-8 breathing to settle your mind before moving into deeper meditative states.

Similarly, incorporating 4-7-8 breathing into your yoga practice can help you stay centered and focused, enhancing the mind-body connection. The rhythmic nature of the breath aligns beautifully with the flow of yoga postures, making it easier to move through your practice with grace and ease.

7. Will this technique help with insomnia, and how long will it take to notice improvements in sleep?

Yes, the 4-7-8 breathing technique is an excellent tool for combating insomnia and improving sleep quality. Many people find that incorporating this technique into their bedtime routine helps to quiet the mind and prepare the body for rest. The deep relaxation induced by the breathing pattern signals to the nervous system that it's time to wind down, making it easier to fall asleep and stay asleep throughout the night.

As for how long it takes to notice improvements, this can vary from person to person. Some individuals experience better sleep after just a few nights of practicing 4-7-8 breathing, while others may need to engage in the practice consistently for a few weeks before seeing significant changes. The key is to remain patient and trust that the cumulative effects of the practice will lead to better sleep over time.

8. Are there any contraindications for practicing the 4-7-8 technique?

While 4-7-8 breathing is safe for most people, those with certain health conditions should approach the practice with caution. If you have a respiratory condition such as asthma, chronic obstructive pulmonary disease (COPD), or other lung issues, it's a good idea to consult with your healthcare provider before starting the practice. The deep, controlled nature of the breath may require adjustments based on your specific condition.

Similarly, if you experience any discomfort, dizziness, or shortness of breath while practicing, it's important to stop and return to your natural breathing rhythm. Everyone's body is different, and what works for one person may need to be modified for another. The goal is always to enhance your well-being, so listen to your body and adjust the practice as needed.

Take a moment to reflect on the information shared in this chapter. Have any of your own questions or concerns been addressed? How might you incorporate the answers provided into your practice of 4-7-8 breathing? Write down any additional questions you have and explore how this technique could continue to evolve in your life.

Conclusion

Throughout this book, you've been guided through the transformative power of the 4-7-8 breathing technique. You've explored the science behind breathwork, learned the step-by-step process, and discovered how this practice can reduce anxiety, improve sleep, enhance focus, and offer a multitude of health benefits. As you've journeyed through these chapters, the goal has been to empower you with the knowledge and tools to cultivate a practice that fits into your life, one that can truly make a difference in your mental and physical well-being.

Here's a brief recap of the essential lessons you've learned:

- **The Power of Breath**: Breathing isn't just a mechanical process; it's a gateway to calm, focus, and healing. By harnessing the breath consciously through techniques like 4-7-8, you can directly influence your nervous system, reduce stress, and cultivate a deeper connection between your mind and body.
- **4-7-8 Breathing Technique**: This simple yet powerful method involves inhaling for 4 counts, holding the breath for 7 counts, and exhaling for 8 counts. Practiced consistently, it can help regulate your emotions, bring clarity to your thoughts, and create a sense of peace, whether you're dealing with momentary stress or chronic anxiety.
- **Application in Daily Life**: From improving sleep to enhancing concentration, 4-7-8 breathing can be incorporated into various aspects of your life. Whether you're lying in bed trying to fall asleep or standing in line

CONCLUSION

at the grocery store, this technique is always available to you as a tool for grounding and balance.
- **Other Health Benefits**: Beyond mental clarity and calmness, this technique offers physical health benefits such as improved digestion, better heart rate variability, and reduced inflammation. It's a holistic practice that can positively affect both your body and mind.
- **Personalized Practice**: No two journeys are the same. Whether you practice once a day or multiple times, whether you find immediate relief or gradual change, this technique can adapt to meet your unique needs. The key is consistency and patience as you allow the practice to unfold naturally in your life.

The 4-7-8 breathing technique is more than just a quick fix—it's a lifelong tool for managing stress, finding balance, and cultivating inner peace. Like any skill, it deepens with practice. Some days, the results may feel subtle, while on other days, the shift may be profound. Through it all, know that every breath you take in this conscious, deliberate way is a step towards greater well-being.

You are on a journey, and this technique is just one part of the path. Continue to practice regularly, even on days when it feels difficult. The more you engage with 4-7-8 breathing, the more natural it will become, and the more benefits you will experience. It may not always be easy, but it will always be worth it.

Remember that change, especially when it comes to something as complex as our mental and physical well-being, takes time. Allow yourself the space to grow into this practice without judgment or frustration. Trust that each breath, each moment of mindfulness, is contributing to a healthier, calmer, and more focused version of yourself.

You are not alone in this journey. Across the world, countless others are discovering the benefits of breathwork, finding solace in the simplicity of inhaling and exhaling with intention. There's a growing community of individuals who are embracing 4-7-8 breathing as a means of improving their lives, and you are invited to join this movement.

Whether through local mindfulness groups, online forums, or social media communities, there are many ways to connect with others who share your interest in breathwork and well-being. Sharing your experiences, challenges, and successes with others can provide valuable support and encouragement. It can also remind you that, while your journey is personal, it is also part of a collective effort towards greater peace and balance in the world.

Consider connecting with like-minded individuals who are on similar paths. Exchange tips, share stories, and encourage one another to keep practicing. Together, you can create a supportive network that fosters growth, healing, and resilience.

As you close this book, know that the journey of 4-7-8 breathing is just beginning. The knowledge you've gained here is a foundation, but the practice itself is a lifelong exploration. Breathe deeply, breathe consciously, and trust in the power of your breath to guide you towards a calmer, clearer, and more centered life.

Welcome to the community of breathers, and may your journey be filled with peace, focus, and joy.

Appendices

▪️ Additional Resources and Tools

As you continue your journey with the 4-7-8 breathing technique, you may find that you want to dive deeper into related practices, learn more about the science behind breathwork, or access tools that can help you stay consistent in your practice. This appendix provides additional resources, including recommended books, apps, and tools to enhance your experience. Whether you're looking to expand your knowledge, stay motivated, or simply track your progress, these resources are designed to support you every step of the way.

<u>Additional Resources</u>

Books on Breathwork and Mindfulness:

- *Breath: The New Science of a Lost Art* by James Nestor: This best-selling book explores the science and history of breathing, offering fascinating insights into how changing the way we breathe can transform our health.
- *The Healing Power of the Breath* by Richard P. Brown, MD, and Patricia L. Gerbarg, MD: A practical guide to breathing techniques that help manage stress, anxiety, and other emotional challenges.
- *Breathe: A Life in Flow* by Rickson Gracie: Written by the legendary Brazilian Jiu-Jitsu master, this book dives into the role of breath in martial arts, mental clarity, and overall well-being.

Scientific Studies on Breathwork:

- The Journal of Psychosomatic Research offers peer-reviewed studies on the impact of breathing techniques on mental and physical health.
- *The Neuroscience of Breathing: From Basic Rhythm to Emotional and Immune Regulation* by MD Patricia L. Gerbarg and PhD Richard P. Brown: This book details the scientific underpinnings of breathwork's influence on the brain and body.

Online Courses and Workshops:

- **Breathing.com**: Offers online courses and resources for mastering various breathing techniques, including the 4-7-8 method.
- **Mindful Schools**: Provides training and resources on mindfulness practices, including breathwork, designed to support educators, parents, and individuals interested in integrating mindfulness into their daily lives.

Videos and Guided Practices:

- **YouTube Channels**: Many experts and practitioners offer free guided breathing exercises, including 4-7-8 breathing, on platforms like YouTube. Look for channels dedicated to mindfulness, yoga, and meditation.
- **Podcasts**: Podcasts like *On Being* with Krista Tippett and *The Daily Meditation Podcast* often feature discussions and guided exercises related to breathwork and mindfulness practices.

Recommended Tools and Applications

Breathing Apps:

- **Calm**: Known for its soothing guided meditations, Calm also includes breathwork exercises that can help you incorporate 4-7-8 breathing into

your daily routine.
- **Breathe2Relax**: A stress management tool that provides guided breathing exercises, including customizable breathing patterns like the 4-7-8 technique.
- **Breathwrk**: This app offers a library of guided breathing exercises designed to help you manage stress, improve focus, and enhance sleep quality.

Mindfulness and Meditation Apps:

- **Headspace**: An app that focuses on meditation and mindfulness but includes breathwork exercises as part of its offerings. It's a great tool for both beginners and seasoned practitioners.
- **Insight Timer**: A popular app with thousands of free guided meditations and breathing exercises. It also allows users to create custom timers for breathwork practices.
- **Oak – Meditation & Breathing**: A simple yet effective app that offers guided breathwork exercises alongside meditation and mindfulness practices. It's perfect for those who prefer an uncluttered, user-friendly experience.

Wearable Devices:

- **Oura Ring**: This wearable tracks sleep patterns, heart rate variability, and other health metrics, helping you understand how your breathwork practice influences your overall well-being.
- **Fitbit**: While primarily a fitness tracker, Fitbit also offers guided breathing sessions and tracks your heart rate, making it a valuable tool for monitoring the effects of your 4-7-8 breathing practice.
- **Spire**: A wearable device designed specifically to monitor your breathing patterns, helping you stay mindful of your breath throughout the day and

encouraging regular practice

Journals and Logs:

- **Daily Wellness Journal**: Keeping a journal can help you track your progress, document your experiences, and reflect on the changes you notice as you incorporate 4-7-8 breathing into your routine.
- **Habit Tracking Apps**: Apps like *HabitBull* or *Streaks* allow you to track your daily breathwork sessions, helping you stay consistent and celebrate your progress.

Community Resources
Online Forums and Groups:

- **Reddit Communities**: Subreddits like r/Meditation, r/Breathwork, and r/Anxiety are great places to connect with others practicing 4-7-8 breathing and similar techniques. You'll find support, advice, and shared experiences from individuals worldwide.
- **Facebook Groups**: Many mindfulness and breathwork communities exist on Facebook, offering a place to share tips, ask questions, and connect with like-minded individuals.

Local Meetups and Classes:

- **Meetup.com**: Search for local meditation and breathwork groups in your area. Practicing with others can enhance your experience and keep you motivated.
- **Yoga and Wellness Studios**: Many studios offer breathwork classes as part of their regular programming. Check out yoga studios, wellness centers, or meditation groups near you to find a community that supports your

practice.

References

📖 Bibliography

In crafting this book, a range of sources have been drawn upon to provide accurate and insightful information on the 4-7-8 breathing technique, its origins, benefits, and applications. Below is a list of key references and further reading for those interested in exploring the topic more deeply.

Books

Brown, Richard P., MD, & Gerbarg, Patricia L., MD. The Healing Power of the Breath: Simple Techniques to Reduce Stress and Anxiety, Enhance Concentration, and Balance Your Emotions. Shambhala, 2012.

Gracie, Rickson. Breathe: A Life in Flow. Dey Street Books, 2021.

Nestor, James. Breath: The New Science of a Lost Art. Riverhead Books, 2020.

Articles and Journals

Brown, Richard P., & Gerbarg, Patricia L. "Yoga Breathing, Meditation, and Longevity." Annals of the New York Academy of Sciences, vol. 1172, no. 1, 2009, pp. 54-62.

Jerath, R., et al. "Physiology of Long Pranayamic Breathing: Neural Respiratory Elements May Provide a Mechanism That Explains How Slow Deep Breathing Shifts the Autonomic Nervous System." Medical Hypotheses, vol. 67, no. 3, 2006, pp. 566-571.

REFERENCES

Telles, Shirley, et al. "Effect of Yoga and Meditation on Sympathetic Nervous System Activity and Cardio-Respiratory Rhythms in Patients with Hypertension." Psychiatry and Clinical Neurosciences, vol. 51, no. 1, 1997, pp. 123-128.

Scientific Studies

Gerbarg, Patricia L., & Brown, Richard P. "Neurobiology of Respiration, Mind-Body Practices and Biobehavioral Regulation." Comprehensive Physiology, vol. 6, no. 4, 2016, pp. 1629-1653.

van Dixhoorn, Jan, & White, Andrew R. "Relaxation Therapy for Rehabilitation and Prevention in Ischemic Heart Disease: A Systematic Review and Meta-analysis." European Journal of Cardiovascular Prevention & Rehabilitation, vol. 12, no. 3, 2005, pp. 193-202.

Online Resources

Harvard Health Publishing. "Yoga for Anxiety and Depression." Harvard Medical School, 2020. https://www.health.harvard.edu/mind-and-mood/yoga-for-anxiety-and-depression

American Psychological Association. "How Stress Affects Your Health." https://www.apa.org/news/press/releases/stress/2019/health-effects

Telles, Shirley, & Singh, Nilkamal. "Science of Breath: Neurophysiological Evidence." International Symposium on Yogism, 2019. Available at https://www.ncbi.nlm.nih.gov.

Research Papers

Peng, C.-K., et al. "Nonlinear Dynamics of Respiratory Patterns in Humans." Journal of Applied Physiology, vol. 95, no. 2, 2003, pp. 107-119.

Streeter, C. C., et al. "Effects of Yoga on the Autonomic Nervous System, Gamma-Aminobutyric-Acid, and Allostasis in Epilepsy, Depression, and Post-Traumatic Stress Disorder." Medical Hypotheses, vol. 78, no. 5, 2012, pp. 571-579.

Milton Keynes UK
Ingram Content Group UK Ltd.
UKHW032048231124
451423UK00013B/1229